Interstitial Cystitis Diet for Women

A Beginner's 3-Step Quick Start Guide to Managing IC Through Diet, With Sample Curated Recipes

mf

copyright © 2022 Mary Golanna

All rights reserved No part of this book may be reproduced, or stored in a retrieval system, or transmitted in any form or by any means, electronic, mechanical, photocopying, recording, or otherwise, without express written permission of the publisher.

Disclaimer

By reading this disclaimer, you are accepting the terms of the disclaimer in full. If you disagree with this disclaimer, please do not read the guide.

All of the content within this guide is provided for informational and educational purposes only, and should not be accepted as independent medical or other professional advice. The author is not a doctor, physician, nurse, mental health provider, or registered nutritionist/dietician. Therefore, using and reading this guide does not establish any form of a physician-patient relationship.

Always consult with a physician or another qualified health provider with any issues or questions you might have regarding any sort of medical condition. Do not ever disregard any qualified professional medical advice or delay seeking that advice because of anything you have read in this guide. The information in this guide is not intended to be any sort of medical advice and should not be used in lieu of any medical advice by a licensed and qualified medical professional.

The information in this guide has been compiled from a variety of known sources. However, the author cannot attest to or guarantee the accuracy of each source and thus should not be held liable for any errors or omissions.

You acknowledge that the publisher of this guide will not be held liable for any loss or damage of any kind incurred as a result of this guide or the reliance on any information provided within this guide. You acknowledge and agree that you assume all risk and responsibility for any action you undertake in response to the information in this guide.

Using this guide does not guarantee any particular result (e.g., weight loss or a cure). By reading this guide, you acknowledge that there are no guarantees to any specific outcome or results you can expect.

All product names, diet plans, or names used in this guide are for identification purposes only and are the property of their respective owners. The use of these names does not imply endorsement. All other trademarks cited herein are the property of their respective owners.

Where applicable, this guide is not intended to be a substitute for the original work of this diet plan and is, at most, a supplement to the original work for this diet plan and never a direct substitute. This guide is a personal expression of the facts of that diet plan.

Where applicable, persons shown in the cover images are stock photography models and the publisher has obtained the rights to use the images through license agreements with third-party stock image companies.

Table of Contents

Introduction   7
What Is Interstitial Cystitis?   9
   What are the symptoms of Interstitial Cystitis?   10
   How is Interstitial Cystitis diagnosed?   11
   Interstitial Cystitis Risk Factors   12
Women and Interstitial Cystitis   13
Complications of Interstitial Cystitis   15
   How to Prevent Interstitial Cystitis?   17
   What Are the Medications for Interstitial Cystitis?   21
Natural Remedies and Lifestyle Changes for Interstitial Cystitis   25
Managing IC Through Diet: A 3-Step Guide   28
   Trigger Foods   29
   Foods that may lessen symptoms   33
Elimination Diet Technique   36
   Step 1: The Elimination Phase   36
   Step 2: The Reintroduction Phase   36
   Step 3: The Maintenance Phase   37
Sample Recipes   39
   Baked Flounder   40
   Asian-Themed Macrobiotic Bowl   41
   Chicken Salad   43
   Baked Salmon   44
   Asian Zucchini Salad   45
   Low FODMAP Burger   46
   Stir-Fried Cabbage and Apples   47
   Asparagus and Greens Salad with Tahini and Poppy Seed Dressing   48
   Stir-Fried Cabbage and Apples   49

Roasted Chicken Thighs	50
Arugula and Mushroom Salad	51
Fresh Asparagus Salad	52
Tuna Salad	54
Conclusion	**55**
References and Helpful Links	**57**

Introduction

Interstitial cystitis (IC) or bladder pain syndrome (BPS) is a long-term health problem with the bladder. It is a pain and pressure in the area around the bladder. Some people have symptoms for a long time, more than 6 weeks without infection or any other obvious cause.

The symptoms vary in how bad they are. Some people's symptoms come and go, while for others they stay the same. IC/BPS is not an infection, but it can feel like a bladder infection. When IC/BPS gets bad, it can affect your life and the lives of those you care about. Some people with IC/BPS also have health problems like IBS, fibromyalgia, and other pain syndromes.

There is no one perfect diet for IC/BPS, but there are certain foods and drinks that can trigger symptoms.

In this guide, we will cover the following topics in depth:

- What is interstitial cystitis?
- What causes interstitial cystitis?
- What are the symptoms of interstitial cystitis?

- How is interstitial cystitis diagnosed?
- Interstitial cystitis risk factors.
- Women and interstitial cystitis.
- Complications of interstitial cystitis.
- How to prevent interstitial cystitis?
- What are the medications for interstitial cystitis?
- Natural remedies and lifestyle changes for interstitial cystitis.
- A 3-step guide to managing interstitial cystitis through diet.

We hope you find this guide helpful and informative. So, let's get started!

What Is Interstitial Cystitis?

Interstitial cystitis is a disorder that affects the bladder and can cause a significant amount of discomfort. It belongs to a range of disorders that are collectively referred to as painful bladder syndrome.

The hollow, muscular structure known as the bladder is responsible for storing your urine. It sends a signal to your brain when it is full, telling your brain that it is time for you to urinate. The majority of people will need to urinate as a result of this.

Interstitial cystitis causes these signals to become jumbled, which results in a sensation that you have to pee more frequently and with smaller amounts of urine than the average person does.

Interstitial cystitis is a condition that most commonly affects women and has the potential to have a significant and long-lasting influence on the quality of life of those who suffer from it. Despite the absence of a cure, there are treatments, including drugs, that can help alleviate symptoms.

What are the symptoms of Interstitial Cystitis?

The symptoms of interstitial cystitis can vary from person to person, and may also change over time. If you are experiencing any of these symptoms, it is important to consult with a healthcare provider to determine the best course of treatment.

Pain in the bladder or pelvic area: The pain may be constant or may come and go. It may be mild, moderate, or severe.

An urgent need to urinate: You may feel the need to urinate more frequently than usual. You may also feel the urge to urinate even when your bladder is not full.

Difficulty emptying your bladder: You may have trouble completely emptying your bladder when you go to the bathroom.

Pain during intercourse: You may feel pain during or after intercourse.

Fatigue: You may feel tired or have difficulty sleeping.

These are the most common symptoms of interstitial cystitis. However, other symptoms may also occur. It is best to speak with a healthcare provider to determine the cause of your symptoms.

How is Interstitial Cystitis diagnosed?

Interstitial cystitis is often difficult to diagnose because the symptoms can vary from person to person and can be similar to those of other conditions. There is no single test that can diagnose interstitial cystitis. Instead, the diagnosis is made based on a combination of factors, including:

Medical history: Your doctor will ask about your symptoms and medical history. They may also ask about your family history, as interstitial cystitis is more common in women who have a family member with the condition.

Physical examination: Your doctor will perform a physical examination to look for signs of interstitial cystitis. This may include a pelvic exam to look for inflammation or other abnormalities in the pelvic area.

Urinalysis: A urinalysis is a test that examines your urine for signs of infection, inflammation, or other abnormalities.

Cystoscopy: A cystoscopy is a procedure that uses a thin, lighted tube to look inside the bladder.

Bladder biopsy: A bladder biopsy is a procedure in which a small sample of tissue is taken from the bladder for testing.

Your doctor may also order other tests to rule out other conditions that can cause similar symptoms. These tests may include imaging tests, such as an MRI or CT scan, or a urodynamic test, which assesses how well the bladder is functioning.

Once other conditions have been ruled out, a diagnosis of interstitial cystitis can be made.

Interstitial Cystitis Risk Factors

Certain factors can increase your risk of developing interstitial cystitis. These include:

Age and gender: Interstitial cystitis is most common in women aged 30-50. Interstitial cystitis is more common in women than in men. This is because the condition is often linked to a history of pelvic inflammatory disease, which is more common in women.

Family history: If you have a family member with interstitial cystitis, you may be at increased risk of developing the condition.

Certain health conditions: Conditions that can increase your risk of interstitial cystitis include endometriosis, irritable bowel syndrome, fibromyalgia, and vulvodynia.

Though there is no cure for interstitial cystitis, there are treatments that can help to relieve symptoms and improve quality of life. If you think you may be at risk of developing interstitial cystitis, talk to your doctor about ways to reduce your risk.

Women and Interstitial Cystitis

Women are more likely to be diagnosed with interstitial cystitis than males are. This may be because the illness is connected to particular hormones, such as estrogen. Interstitial cystitis symptoms frequently become more severe around the time of menstruation, which may be due to the fluctuating amounts of estrogen that occur throughout the menstrual cycle.

Alterations in hormone levels can also be brought on by pregnancy, which might bring on symptoms of interstitial cystitis or make them worse. Because giving birth vaginally can cause injury to the muscles and nerves of the pelvic floor, women who have given birth vaginally are also more likely to suffer from interstitial cystitis.

In addition, Kirkham and Swainston authored a qualitative study that was published in the Western Journal of Nursing Research. The study is titled "Women's Experiences of Interstitial Cystitis/Painful Bladder Syndrome," and it discusses the experiences of women who have painful bladder syndrome and interstitial cystitis. The purpose of this qualitative study was to investigate the lived experiences of women who have IC or PBS to have a better understanding of those women's reality. The debilitating ailment known as interstitial cystitis/painful bladder syndrome (IC/PBS) can have a significant and negative influence on the quality of life of women who are affected by it.

According to the findings of the study, the women who were questioned suffered from a broad variety of symptoms, which affected every aspect of their life. Because there are still a lot of stigmas linked to IC/PBS, many people feel lonely and alone because of it. Participants talked about experiencing emotions of helplessness and frustration, and many of them claimed that they did not feel like they had enough assistance from medical personnel.

This study contributes significantly to our understanding of the lived experiences of women who have IC or PBS, and it will assist in guiding and informing future research and treatments in this field.

Complications of Interstitial Cystitis

Interstitial cystitis can cause several complications, such as:

Urinary tract infections: Individuals who have IC have a higher risk of developing urinary tract infections (UTIs). Urinary tract infections are brought on by bacteria that make their way into the urinary system and then multiply there. After reaching the bladder, the germs can create an infection there if they remain there long enough.

Because the lining of the bladder is already inflamed and damaged, those who have IC have a greater risk of developing urinary tract infections (UTIs). Because of this, it is much simpler for bacteria to attach themselves to the wall of the bladder and produce an infection.

Kidney damage: Interstitial cystitis can cause kidney damage if it is allowed to go untreated for an extended period. Infections of the urinary tract are often the root cause of kidney damage brought on by interstitial cystitis. Infections of the urinary tract are possible outcomes of bacteria migrating from the bladder to the kidneys. Early identification and treatment of interstitial cystitis can help avoid damage to the kidneys that can be caused by the condition.

Sexual dysfunction: Interstitial cystitis can cause sexual dysfunction, such as pain during intercourse or an inability to orgasm.

Infertility: Interstitial cystitis is a disorder that can lead to infertility in both men and women. This is because the illness affects the urinary tract. Inflammation of the bladder is a hallmark of this disorder, which, if left untreated, can result in scarring and a blockage of the tubes that transport sperm and eggs.

Interstitial cystitis can also thin the lining of a woman's uterus, making it harder for a fertilized egg to implant in the uterus. This condition only affects women. In males, the illness can result in inflammation of the testicles, which can impede the generation of sperm and induce infertility.

Psychological complication: Interstitial cystitis can cause psychological difficulties such as worry and sadness, in addition to the physical symptoms that are often associated with the condition. Dealing with the ailment can be challenging because of the persistent discomfort and the disruption it causes in one's normal routine. Because of this, a significant number of individuals who have interstitial cystitis also have symptoms of anxiety and sadness.

If they are not addressed, these psychological difficulties might make the disease much more difficult to manage and cause it to deteriorate further. Therefore, getting therapy for both the physical and psychological symptoms of interstitial cystitis is quite crucial.

If left untreated, interstitial cystitis can lead to several complications. These complications can range from mild to severe, and they can have a significant impact on the quality of life of those affected by the condition. Early diagnosis and treatment are essential to prevent these complications from occurring.

How to Prevent Interstitial Cystitis?

There is no sure way to prevent interstitial cystitis. However, there are some things you can do to reduce your risk of developing the condition. These include:

Quit smoking: Interstitial cystitis is more likely to develop in smokers than in non-smokers, and the likelihood of developing the condition rises in proportion to the number of cigarettes smoked daily. Quitting smoking is the single most important step you can take to lower your chances of developing interstitial cystitis.

There are numerous tools available to assist you to succeed in quitting smoking, including counseling, support groups, and medicine, even though quitting may be tough for you. Have a conversation with your primary care physician right away about giving up smoking and dealing with interstitial cystitis.

Manage stress: It is thought that stress may have a role in causing symptoms to manifest themselves or in making them worse. The symptoms of interstitial cystitis tend to become more severe if the patient is under more emotional or physical strain. Learning how to manage stress can help prevent interstitial cystitis from forming or lessen the intensity of symptoms, even though there is currently no treatment that can cure the illness.

Consider speaking with a counselor or your primary care physician if you find that you are unable to cope with the effects of stress. Several different relaxation techniques can assist to lower levels of stress.

Eat a healthy diet: Diet plays a significant part in the management of IC, and maintaining a nutritious diet is critical to one's general health and well-being. Caffeine, artificial sweeteners, alcohol, and very hot meals can all be dietary triggers for irritable bowel syndrome (IC). In addition, a diet that is heavy in acidic foods has been shown in several studies to be associated with an increased likelihood of getting IC.

For this reason, it is essential to maintain a healthy diet that consists of a sufficient quantity of fruits and vegetables. If you want to enhance your general health and lower your chance of developing interstitial cystitis, eating a diet high in healthful foods will help.

Exercise regularly: It is believed that regular exercise can improve IC by alleviating stress in the muscles, boosting circulation to the pelvic region, and enhancing the performance of the muscles in the urinary system. If you have IC, you should discuss the possibility of participating in physical activity with your primary care provider.

Drink plenty of fluids: It is hypothesized that the accumulation of waste items in the urine may play a role in the development of interstitial cystitis. [Citation needed] Consuming a sufficient amount of fluids can assist in the removal of waste items from the body and may lower the likelihood that you will develop interstitial cystitis. In addition, drinking plenty of fluids can assist in the diluting of urine, which in turn makes it less unpleasant to the bladder. If you are at risk of developing interstitial cystitis, it is essential to ensure that you consume a sufficient amount of fluids daily.

Avoid irritants: Caffeine, alcohol, and meals with a spicy flavor are examples of the kinds of things that can irritate the bladder and make the symptoms of interstitial cystitis even worse. It is possible that avoiding these drugs can help prevent the illness from forming or will lessen the intensity of the symptoms if it already exists.

Do not hold your urine: When you feel the need to urinate, it is critical to pay attention to what your body is telling you and act accordingly by going to the restroom. Interstitial cystitis is a disorder that causes pain and inflammation in the bladder. If you hold your pee in for too long, it can irritate the bladder and lead to this ailment. Interstitial cystitis can cause excruciating discomfort, and it may also result in infections of the urinary system. In severe instances, it is even capable of causing damage to the kidneys.

Talk to your doctor: You must consult a medical professional if you are suffering any urinary symptoms, such as discomfort or increased frequency of urination. Early identification and treatment are essential for reducing the severity of symptoms and reducing the risk of consequences. Interstitial cystitis is an illness that can be severe, but many individuals can control their symptoms and lead lives that are reasonably normal after receiving an early diagnosis and the appropriate therapy.

Don't be afraid to consult a medical professional if you notice any symptoms related to your urinary system. The key to avoiding interstitial cystitis from taking over your life is getting a diagnosis and starting therapy as soon as possible.

Interstitial cystitis is a chronic condition that can have a significant impact on your quality of life. There is no cure for interstitial cystitis, but there are treatments that can help to manage symptoms. If you think you may have interstitial cystitis, talk to your doctor.

What Are the Medications for Interstitial Cystitis?

There is no one-size-fits-all approach to treating interstitial cystitis. The best course of treatment will depend on the individual and the severity of their symptoms. Medications that may be used to treat interstitial cystitis include:

Antibiotics: If you have IC, your doctor will likely recommend a course of antibiotic therapy if they believe an infection is present. Antibiotic therapy is usually effective in treating IC, but it is important to finish the full course of treatment to prevent recurrent infections.

Pain relief medication: Over-the-counter and prescription pain medications may help to manage the associated pain. The most common type of pain relief medication used for interstitial cystitis is an analgesic, which can help to reduce inflammation and provide relief from discomfort.

In some cases, a combination of medications may be necessary to achieve optimal pain relief. When exploring different options for pain management, it is important to discuss possible side effects with a doctor.

Bladder instillations: Bladder instillations are a type of therapy that involves placing medication directly into the bladder. This treatment can help to reduce inflammation and pain associated with interstitial cystitis. Bladder instillations are usually done in a doctor's office or outpatient clinic. The doctor will insert a catheter into the bladder and then infuse the medication through the catheter.

The medication is typically held in the bladder for 20-30 minutes before being drained. Bladder instillations are usually done once or twice a week for several weeks. This treatment can be effective in reducing symptoms of interstitial cystitis. It is important to talk to your doctor about any potential side effects of this therapy before starting treatment.

Muscle relaxants: Muscle relaxants may help to relieve some of these symptoms by reducing the muscle spasms in the bladder. There are a variety of muscle relaxants that can be used for this purpose, and your doctor will work with you to choose the best one for you. In some cases, muscle relaxants may need to be taken regularly to help keep the muscle spasms under control.

Tricyclic antidepressants: Tricyclic antidepressants are a type of medication that is commonly used to treat conditions like interstitial cystitis. Tricyclic antidepressants work by blocking the reuptake of certain neurotransmitters, which helps to improve pain and sleep. Tricyclic antidepressants can help to reduce urinary frequency and urgency and improve sleep quality in people with interstitial cystitis. If you are considering taking tricyclic antidepressants for your interstitial cystitis, be sure to talk to your doctor about the potential risks and benefits.

Pentosan polysulfate: Pentosan polysulfate works by binding to the bladder wall, which helps to protect it from irritants. It also helps to reduce inflammation and pain by inhibiting the production of inflammatory mediators. In addition, pentosan polysulfate helps to increase the amount of mucus in the bladder, which provides a barrier against irritants.

Pentosan polysulfate is typically taken orally, although it can also be given rectally or intravesically. The most common side effects of pentosan polysulfate are urinary frequency, urgency, and dysuria. Less common side effects include constipation, gastrointestinal upset, and skin rash.

Botulinum toxin: Botulinum toxin injections can help to reduce muscle spasms and provide relief from IC symptoms. The injections work by temporarily paralyzing the muscles, which helps to reduce spasms and pain. In addition, the injections can help to improve bladder function and prevent urinary leakage. For many people with IC, botulinum toxin injections are an essential part of managing their condition and improving their quality of life.

Surgery: Surgery may be an option for some people with interstitial cystitis. Surgery is typically only considered when other treatment options have failed.

Important to note: These are just some of the medications that may be used to treat interstitial cystitis. The best course of treatment will vary from person to person. It is important to discuss all of your treatment options with your doctor.

Natural Remedies and Lifestyle Changes for Interstitial Cystitis

In addition to medication, several natural remedies and lifestyle changes can help to manage interstitial cystitis symptoms. These include:

Dietary changes: There are several treatments available for IC, but avoiding triggering foods and beverages is often the first line of defense. Caffeine, alcohol, and spicy foods can all irritate the bladder and exacerbate IC symptoms. In addition, some people find that acidic foods, such as tomatoes and citrus fruits, also trigger symptoms. By avoiding these trigger foods and drinks, you may be able to reduce your IC symptoms.

Stress reduction: When we experience stress, our bodies produce the hormone cortisol, which can cause inflammation in the bladder. In addition, stress can lead to muscle tension and pain in the pelvic region. By taking steps to manage stress, we can help to reduce the frequency and severity of IC symptoms.

There are many different ways to do this, such as relaxation therapy and yoga. If you suffer from IC, experiment with different stress-management methods to see what works best for you.

Exercise: Exercise can help to relieve some of the symptoms of IC. Exercise helps to increase blood flow to the pelvis, which can help to reduce pain. In addition, exercise helps to reduce stress levels, which can also help to reduce pain and promote overall health. While there is no cure for IC, exercise can help to make living with the condition easier.

Acupuncture: Acupuncture is a type of alternative therapy that involves placing needles in the skin. It is based on the belief that there are unseen energy pathways (or "meridians") that run throughout the body, and that disruptions in these meridians can cause disease. By placing needles at specific points along these pathways, practitioners believe that they can restore balance and improve health.

Bladder training: Bladder training involves gradually increasing the amount of time between urination. This can help to retrain the bladder and reduce frequency and urgency. IC is a complex condition, and bladder training is not a cure. However, it may help to improve symptoms and quality of life.

While there is no exact cure for interstitial cystitis, the condition can be managed with medication, natural remedies, and lifestyle changes. If you think you may have interstitial cystitis, talk to your doctor. Early diagnosis and treatment are important for preventing complications and managing symptoms.

Managing IC Through Diet: A 3-Step Guide

If you have interstitial cystitis, you may be looking for ways to manage your symptoms. Diet can play an important role in managing IC. Here is a 3-step guide to getting started:

Step 1: Avoid foods and beverages that can irritate the bladder. People with IC often find that certain foods and beverages can irritate their bladder, exacerbating their symptoms. In general, acidic foods and drinks, spicy dishes, caffeine, and alcohol should be avoided. However, every individual is different, so it's important to pay attention to your own body and identify which foods trigger your symptoms. Once you know which foods to avoid, you can make adjustments to your diet that will help you manage your IC.

Step 2: Eat a healthy diet. A healthy diet is important for everyone, but it's especially crucial for people with IC. A diet that's high in fiber and low in sodium can help to reduce bladder irritation and minimize symptoms. Eating plenty of fruits, vegetables, and whole grains is a good way to ensure that you're getting the fiber you need while avoiding processed foods will help keep your sodium intake in check.

Step 3: Drink plenty of fluids. It's important to stay hydrated when you have IC, as dehydration can irritate the bladder and make symptoms worse. Aim to drink eight glasses of water or other non-caffeinated beverages each day. If you find it difficult to drink that much fluid, try spreading it out throughout the day or drinking smaller amounts more frequently. You may also want to try adding mint leaves to your water to give it a flavor without using any irritating ingredients.

Making these dietary changes can help to reduce IC symptoms and improve your quality of life. Talk to your doctor about other ways to manage IC.

Trigger Foods

Citrus Fruits: Citrus fruits are thought to be one of the trigger foods for people with interstitial cystitis, due to their high acid content. When citrus fruits are consumed, the acid can irritate the bladder lining, causing inflammation and pain. IC sufferers should avoid citrus fruits, or consume them in small amounts. If you think citrus fruits may be triggering your IC symptoms, talk to your doctor or dietitian about ways to limit their impact on your condition.

Tomatoes: The acidity of tomatoes can irritate the bladder, leading to discomfort and an urge to urinate more frequently. Some people with interstitial cystitis find that avoiding tomatoes helps to reduce their symptoms. If you're struggling with this condition, it may be worth eliminating tomatoes from your diet to see if it makes a difference.

However, everyone is different, and some people with interstitial cystitis can tolerate tomatoes without any problems. If you're not sure whether tomatoes are a trigger food for you, it's best to speak to a doctor or dietitian who can help you figure out an eating plan that will minimize your symptoms.

Chocolate: Chocolate contains compounds that can irritate the bladder, triggering IC symptoms. In addition, chocolate also contains caffeine and theobromine, two stimulants that can increase urinary frequency. For these reasons, people with IC should avoid chocolate and other potential triggers, such as spicy foods, carbonated beverages, and artificial sweeteners. By doing so, they may be able to minimize their symptoms and enjoy a better quality of life.

Coffee: Coffee contains compounds that can irritate the bladder, and it is also a diuretic, which can increase urinary frequency. In addition, coffee has been shown to increase inflammation in the body, which may contribute to pain and other IC symptoms. If you suspect that coffee is triggering your IC symptoms, you may want to try eliminating it from your diet for some time to see if your symptoms improve.

Spicy Foods: Spicy foods are believed to trigger the symptoms of interstitial cystitis. When capsaicin, the compound that gives chili peppers their heat, comes into contact with the bladder, it can cause irritation and pain. In addition, capsaicin may increase the release of the substance P, a chemical involved in pain signals.

If you suffer from interstitial cystitis, you may want to avoid spicy foods or use them sparingly. You should also drink plenty of water to help flush out irritants and stay hydrated. By taking these precautions, you can help reduce your symptoms and enjoy your favorite foods without pain.

Dairy: Dairy products contain a type of sugar called lactose, which can be difficult to digest. When lactose isn't properly broken down, it can travel to the bladder, where it can irritate the lining and cause inflammation. In addition, dairy products are a common source of food allergies, and allergic reactions can also contribute to IC flare-ups. If you suspect that dairy is triggering your IC symptoms, you may want to try eliminating it from your diet for a few weeks to see if your symptoms improve.

Alcohol: Alcohol has been shown to increase urinary frequency and urgency. In addition, alcohol can irritate the lining of the bladder, further worsening symptoms. For these reasons, patients with IC should limit their alcohol intake or avoid alcohol altogether.

Processed Foods: Processed foods, in particular, may trigger IC symptoms. These foods are often high in additives and preservatives, which can irritate the bladder and cause inflammation. In addition, processed foods are often high in sugar or artificial sweeteners, which can worsen urinary frequency and urgency. If you suspect that processed foods are triggering your IC symptoms, eliminating them from your diet may help to improve your health.

Onions: Onions contain compounds that can be irritating to the bladder, and they are also high in sulfur, which can increase urine acidity. For people with IC, onions can exacerbate symptoms such as frequency and urgency. In some cases, they may also lead to bladder spasms, which can be extremely painful. If you have IC, it's important to pay attention to your diet and avoid triggering foods like onions.

Gluten: Gluten is a protein found in wheat, rye, and barley, and when it comes into contact with the bladder, it can cause inflammation and irritation. For women with IC, this can lead to increased pelvic pain and urinary frequency. While more research is needed to confirm the link between gluten and IC, avoiding gluten may help to relieve symptoms in some women.

Artificial sweeteners: Artificial sweeteners are thought to trigger the symptoms of interstitial cystitis by altering the composition of the gut microbiota. This changes the way the body breaks down and eliminates waste, leading to inflammation of the bladder. If you are seeking relief from interstitial cystitis, it is best to avoid artificial sweeteners and other potential triggers, such as caffeine and spicy foods. With proper management, interstitial cystitis can be a manageable condition.

Foods that may lessen symptoms

Water: By staying hydrated, patients can flush out any irritants that may be causing inflammation. In addition, water helps to dilute the urine and reduce the frequency of urinary urgency. As a result, drinking six to eight glasses of water each day can be an effective way to manage interstitial cystitis. Of course, everyone's needs are different, so it's important to talk to a doctor about the best way to manage this condition.

Garlic: Garlic is thought to be beneficial for interstitial cystitis because it contains a compound called allicin, which has anti-inflammatory and antimicrobial properties. In addition, garlic is a natural diuretic, which can help to flush out the bladder and reduce urinary frequency. While more research is needed to definitively prove that garlic can help ease the symptoms of interstitial cystitis, it is safe to say that this potent little herb has many potential health benefits.

Turmeric: Turmeric contains a compound called curcumin, which has been shown to have anti-inflammatory properties. Curcumin is thought to work by inhibiting the activity of certain immune system cells. This action may help to reduce inflammation in the bladder and relieve the symptoms of interstitial cystitis.

Leafy green vegetables: Leafy green vegetables are a natural source of compounds that may help to lessen the symptoms of interstitial cystitis. For example, the nutrients in leafy greens can help to reduce inflammation and improve urinary function. In addition, the high water content of leafy greens can help to flush out irritants from the bladder. While there is no cure for interstitial cystitis, incorporating leafy green vegetables into your diet may help to ease your symptoms.

Chamomile tea: Chamomile tea is brewed using the dried flowers of the plant Camellia sinensis. This herbal tea has been used for centuries to treat a variety of ailments, including indigestion, anxiety, and insomnia. Chamomile tea contains compounds that have anti-inflammatory and antimicrobial properties.

In addition, chamomile tea is a rich source of flavonoids, which are plant-based antioxidants that help to protect cells from damage. A cup of chamomile tea can help to lessen the symptoms of IC by reducing inflammation and promoting healing.

Elimination Diet Technique

If you're not sure which foods or beverages are irritating your bladder, you may want to try an elimination diet. This involves removing potential irritants from your diet for some time and then slowly reintroducing them one at a time. This can help you to identify which foods or beverages are triggering your IC symptoms.

Step 1: The Elimination Phase

The first step in the elimination phase is to cut out all potential trigger foods from your diet. The goal of this phase is to help you identify which foods may be causing your symptoms. Once you've eliminated all potential trigger foods from your diet, you'll need to carefully monitor your symptoms for some time. If your symptoms improve during this phase, one or more of the eliminated foods was likely contributing to your symptoms.

Step 2: The Reintroduction Phase

The reintroduction phase is an important part of the process. Once you have identified your trigger foods, you can begin to reintroduce them one at a time. This will help you figure out how much of each food you can tolerate without experiencing symptoms. The key is to go slowly and to pay attention to your body. You may find that some foods are more tolerable than others, and that's okay. The goal is to find a balance that works for you.

And remember, if you do experience symptoms, it's important to back off and give your body a break. With a little trial and error, you'll be on your way to finding the perfect diet for your unique needs.

Step 3: The Maintenance Phase

In the maintenance phase, it's important to continue following the diet that you found to be the most helpful in the reintroduction phase. You may need to make some adjustments to this diet as your symptoms change over time.

It's also important to eat regularly and include a variety of nutrient-rich foods in your diet to ensure you're getting all the nutrients your body needs. Some people find it helpful to keep a food diary during this phase so they can track their symptoms and figure out what foods trigger their symptoms. If you find that your symptoms are getting worse or you're having difficulty sticking to the diet, it's important to talk to a Registered Dietitian or another healthcare professional for help.

By following these steps, you can develop an IC diet that works for you. Just remember to work with a doctor or dietitian to make sure that you're getting all the nutrients you need while still avoiding your trigger foods.

Sample Recipes

Baked Flounder

Ingredients:

- 1 lb. flounder, fileted
- 1/4 tsp. salt
- 1 cup halved red grapes
- 1 tbsp. extra-virgin olive oil
- 2 tbsp. parsley, chopped finely
- 1 cup almonds, chopped and toasted
- freshly ground black pepper, to taste

Instructions:

1. Preheat the oven to 375°F.
2. Place fish on a sheet tray. Season with olive oil, salt, and pepper.
3. Combine the almonds, grapes, parsley, 1-1/2 tsp. of olive oil, 1/8 tsp of salt, and black pepper in a bowl.
4. Bake the fish for about 3 minutes.
5. Flip the fish and return to the oven.
6. Bake for another 3 minutes, or until the fish is starting to flake, while the center is still translucent. Don't overcook.
7. Serve immediately, topped with the grape mixture.

Asian-Themed Macrobiotic Bowl

Ingredients:

- 2 cups cooked quinoa
- 4 carrots
- 1 package of smoked tofu
- 1 tbsp. nutritional yeast
- 2 tbsp. coconut aminos
- 4 tbsp. sunflower sprouts
- 2 tbsp. fermented vegetables
- 1 cup of shiitake mushrooms
- 1 avocado
- 2 tbsp. hemp seeds
- 2-3 cooked beets
- coconut oil cooking spray

Dressing:

- 2 tbsp. miso paste
- 1 tbsp. tahini
- 1 tbsp. olive oil
- 3 tbsp. water

Instructions:

1. Roast the carrots in the oven at 400°F for 30-40 minutes.
2. Wash the vegetables, trim them, and spray them with coconut oil.

3. Add them to the oven. When they are cooked, set aside till you are ready to assemble the Buddha bowl.
4. Make the dressing by combining all of the ingredients in a medium-sized bowl. If the dressing appears lumpy, add more water.
5. To build the bowl, put the quinoa on the bottom and then arrange the vegetables on top.
6. Sprinkle the bowls with hemp seeds and drizzle the dressing over top.
7. Now serve and enjoy

Chicken Salad

Ingredients:

- 1 small can premium chunk chicken breast packed in water
- 1 stalk celery, large, finely chopped
- 1/4 cup reduced-fat mayonnaise
- 4 romaine leaves or red leaf lettuce, washed and trimmed
- 1 cucumber, small and sliced thinly

Instructions:

1. Drain canned chicken and transfer to a bowl.
2. Put in celery and mayonnaise.
3. Mix lightly. Don't crush the chicken.
4. In a separate shallow bowl, place the lettuce neatly.
5. Add the chicken salad in the middle
6. Add cucumber slices to the plate.
7. Refrigerate before serving, cover with plastic wrap.

Baked Salmon

Ingredients:

- 2 salmon filets
- 6 cups of fresh spinach
- 2 tsp. coconut oil
- 1/4 tsp. turmeric
- salt
- pepper

Instructions:

1. Preheat the oven to 400°F.
2. Line a baking dish with parchment paper.
3. Marinate salmon filets coconut oil, turmeric, salt, and pepper.
4. Let it sit for a few minutes. This may also be done the night before to help the juices and flavor get into the salmon.
5. Once the oven is ready, bake the salmon for 15 minutes.
6. Add spinach and cook until ready. Season with salt and pepper to taste.
7. Take salmon out of the oven and put spinach beside it.
8. Serve and enjoy.

Asian Zucchini Salad

Ingredients:

- 1 medium zucchini, sliced thinly into spirals
- 1/3 cup rice vinegar
- 3/4 cup avocado oil
- 1 cup sunflower seeds, shells removed
- 1 lb. cabbage, shredded
- 1 tsp. stevia drops
- 1 cup almonds, sliced

Instructions:

1. Cut the zucchini spirals into smaller parts. Set aside.
2. Put almonds, sunflower seeds, and cabbage in a large bowl. Combine the ingredients well.
3. Add zucchini to the mixture.
4. In a small bowl, mix vinegar, stevia, and oil using a whisk or fork.
5. Pour the vinegar mixture all over the zucchini mixture. Toss well. Make sure everything is covered with the dressing.
6. Refrigerate for 2 hours before serving.

Low FODMAP Burger

Ingredients:

- 1-1/4 lbs. ground pork
- 1/2 tsp. salt
- 1/2 tsp. white pepper
- 1/2 tsp. ground nutmeg
- 1/2 tsp. caraway seeds
- 1/2 tsp. ground ginger

Instructions:

1. Preheat the grill then prepare the patty.
2. Using a small mixing bowl, stir together the salt, pepper, nutmeg, and ginger until fully combined.
3. Place the ground in a large mixing bowl and add the spice mixture.
4. Mix thoroughly until spices are evenly distributed to the pork.
5. Make round, flat burger patties using the palm of your hands.
6. Grill the patties and serve with gluten-free buns and mustard sauce.

Stir-Fried Cabbage and Apples

Ingredients:

- 1 shallot, thinly sliced
- 1/2 apple, cut into cubes
- 1/4 savoy cabbage, sliced thinly into strips
- 3–4 radishes, sliced thinly
- 1/2–1 tsp. coconut oil
- salt, to taste

Instructions:

1. Pour some coconut oil into a wok.
2. Add shallot and cook until translucent.
3. Add the cabbage, radish, and apples to the wok.
4. Stir-fry for about 5 minutes. Don't overcook.
5. Add salt to taste.
6. Serve while warm.

Asparagus and Greens Salad with Tahini and Poppy Seed Dressing

Ingredients:

- 10 to 12 asparagus stalks, washed well and sliced into ribbons
- 5 radishes, washed well, and sliced thinly
- 2 to 3 rainbow carrots, peeled and sliced thinly
- 1 handful wild spinach
- 1 small handful of microgreens, washed well
- 1 small handful of sunflower greens, washed well
- optional: few pieces of chive blossoms

For the dressing:

- 2 tbsp. tahini
- 1 tbsp. poppy seeds
- 1 tbsp. extra-virgin olive oil
- salt
- pepper

Instructions:

1. For the dressing, whisk ingredients together in a small bowl.
2. In a separate bowl, toss salad ingredients in the mixture.
3. Drizzle dressing on salad upon serving.

Stir-Fried Cabbage and Apples

Ingredients:

- 1 shallot, thinly sliced
- 1/2 apple, cut into cubes
- 1/4 savoy cabbage, sliced thinly into strips
- 3–4 radishes, sliced thinly
- 1/2–1 tsp. coconut oil
- salt, to taste

Instructions:

1. Pour some coconut oil into a wok.
2. Add shallot and cook until translucent.
3. Add the cabbage, radish, and apples to the wok.
4. Stir-fry for about 5 minutes. Don't overcook.
5. Add salt to taste.
6. Serve while warm.

Roasted Chicken Thighs

Ingredients:

- 1 tbsp. avocado oil
- 1 pinch Himalayan pink salt
- 4 chicken thighs with skin
- 1 tsp. Primal Palate super gyro seasoning

Instructions:

1. Pour avocado oil over a medium-sized oven-safe pot.
2. Sauté over medium heat for 2 to 3 minutes or until the skins begin to brown.
3. Place the chicken in a large skillet over medium-high heat. Sear for about 2 to 3 minutes for each side, starting with the skin side.
4. Season generously with salt and Primal Palate Super Gyro seasoning.
5. Place the chicken in an oven preheated to 350°F.
6. Bake for one hour while covered.
7. Serve and enjoy.

Arugula and Mushroom Salad

Ingredients:

- 5 oz. arugula washed
- 1 lb. fresh mushrooms
- 1/4 tsp. shoyu
- 1 tbsp. olive oil
- 1 tbsp. mirin

For tofu cheese:

- 1/8 cup umeboshi vinegar
- 1/2 firm tofu

Instructions:

1. In a bowl, add the rinsed tofu. Crumble and pour in vinegar.
2. In a separate bowl add shoyu, salt, olive oil, and mirin. 3. Mix to combine.
3. Add in the arugula and toss to combine with the dressing.
4. Serve and enjoy.

Fresh Asparagus Salad

Ingredients:

- 1/3 cup of hazelnuts
- 4 cups arugula
- 1 tsp. ground pepper
- 2 tbsp. sea salt
- virgin olive oil
- 2 lbs. asparagus

Instructions:

1. Preheat the oven to 400°F.
2. Place hazelnuts on a baking tray with parchment paper. Place in the oven for 7 minutes.
3. Transfer hazelnuts to a plate. Optionally, to remove the skins, wrap the nuts in a towel and rub them vigorously.
4. Chop hazelnuts coarsely.
5. Remove the hard ends of the asparagus.
6. Place the stalks on the baking sheet you've used for the hazelnuts. Sprinkle 1 tbsp. olive oil and 1/2 tsp. of salt.
7. Bake for 8 minutes.
8. In a mixing bowl, combine pepper, salt, and olive oil. Mix well.

9. Place arugula in a medium bowl. Drizzle ½ of the dressing over the veggies. Toss until everything is well coated.
10. Place arugula onto a platter.
11. Arrange asparagus on top. Sprinkle peeled hazelnuts on top.

Tuna Salad

Ingredients:

- 1/2 cup pecans
- 1 cup chicken breast, steamed and cubed
- 1 cup tuna in oil
- salt, to taste
- pepper, to taste

Instructions:

1. Mix all ingredients in a large bowl.
2. Add a dash of salt and pepper to taste.
3. Chill for at least an hour before serving.

Conclusion

The condition known as interstitial cystitis (IC) affects the bladder and causes discomfort and irritation. It is not understood exactly what causes IC, but experts suspect that an autoimmune reaction may be to blame. It appears to have a hereditary basis since it is seen to be more prevalent in females than in males. Certain health disorders, age, gender, and history of the illness in the family are among the risk factors for IC.

Pain in the bladder and pelvic region, urinary urgency and frequency, and burning sensations during urination are the most common symptoms of interstitial cystitis (IC), however, these symptoms can vary widely from person to person. A combination of the patient's symptoms, their medical history, and the results of laboratory testing are used to arrive at a diagnosis of IC. No treatment is guaranteed to work for everyone who has IC; however, some popular therapies include drugs, bladder injections, physical therapy, and dietary changes.

Dietary management of inflammatory bowel disease (IC) might be difficult at times, but it is not impossible with some hard work. The first thing that should be done is to cut out any items that are known to make the disease worse. The second stage is to gradually reintroduce those foods one by one to see which ones produce the least amount of distress. The third stage is to develop an individualized eating strategy that is tailored to your requirements.

If you follow these measures, you will have a better chance of managing your IC and improving the quality of your life.

References and Helpful Links

Abedin, S. (n.d.). Interstitial cystitis. WebMD. Retrieved October 16, 2022, from
https://www.webmd.com/urinary-incontinence-oab/interstitial-cystitis.

Bladder irritating foods: Symptoms & diet i atlanta, ga. (n.d.). Https://Ugatl.Com/. Retrieved October 16, 2022, from https://ugatl.com/services/overactive-bladder/foods-that-irritate-the-bladder-and-urethra/.

Foods to avoid | Interstitial Cystitis Association. (2021, October 7). https://www.ichelp.org/understanding-ic/diet/foods-to-avoid/.

Hooker, J. (2021, July 19). Interstitial cystitis diet: What to eat & what to avoid - primehealth denver. https://primehealthdenver.com/interstitial-cystitis-diet/.

How to follow the interstitial cystitis diet. (2022, May 23). Healthline. https://www.healthline.com/nutrition/interstitial-cystitis-diet.

Interstitial cystitis—Symptoms and causes. (n.d.). Mayo Clinic. Retrieved October 16, 2022, from https://www.mayoclinic.org/diseases-conditions/interstitial-cystitis/symptoms-causes/syc-20354357.

Kirkham, A., & Swainston, K. (2022). Women's experiences of interstitial cystitis/painful bladder syndrome. Western Journal of Nursing Research, 44(2), 125–132. https://doi.org/10.1177/0193945921990730.

Ridouh, I., & Hackshaw, K. V. (2022). Essential oils and neuropathic pain. Plants, 11(14), 1797. https://doi.org/10.3390/plants11141797.

What is interstitial cystitis(Ic)/bladder pain syndrome? - Urology care foundation. (n.d.). Retrieved October 16, 2022, from https://www.urologyhealth.org/urology-a-z/i/interstitial-cystitis.

www.ingramcontent.com/pod-product-compliance
Lightning Source LLC
LaVergne TN
LVHW011859060526
838200LV00054B/4422